Lose Weight Naturally

from the
Naturally Simple Health Series

by

Stephanie Yeh

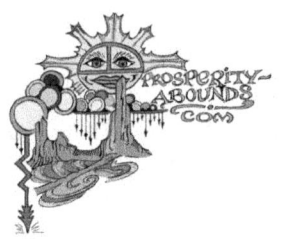

Contact Information: syeh@stephanieyeh.com
Visit my website: www.prosperity-abounds.com

Disclaimer and Legal Notice:

Lose Weight Naturally

Simple Strategies | Healthy Options

From the Naturally Simple Health Series

by Stephanie Yeh

Table of Contents

Lose Weight Naturally

√ Simple Strategies
√ Healthy Options

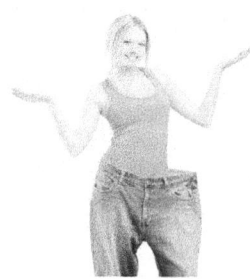

Eat half a grapefruit before meals to lose as much as one pound per week, since grapefruit lowers the hormone (insulin) for fat storage.
(National Institutes of Health)

Add intense periods of exercise during moderate exercise, such as adding bursts of jogging during a walk, to burn more calories.
(The American College of Sports Medicine)

Take enzymes between meals... enzymes will "scavenge" throughout your body and help flush toxins, which can increase weight loss.

Practice carb cycling. Alternate high and low-carb days, with heavier exercise on high-carb days.

Take high-quality probiotic supplements, which block fat absorption, help the body rid itself of fat, and prevent fat storage.
(National Institutes of Health)

Do resistance exercises. Any resistance training, such as weight lifting, will help build lean muscle, which burns more calories than other types of tissue. Resistance exercise helps prevent the loss of muscle mass while dieting.
(WebMD)

Is This You?

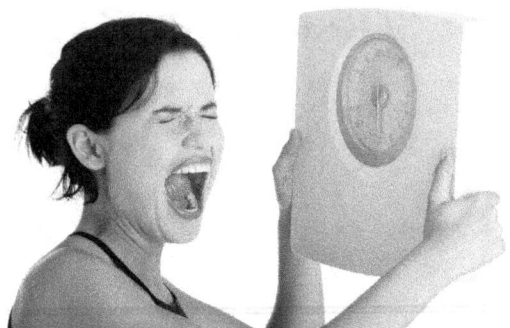

You are **NOT** alone!

Did You Know That ...

- **2 out of 3 adults in the U.S. are overweight or obese.**
  (National Health and Nutrition Examination Survey, 2009–2010)

- **50% of women who have lost weight report that they gain it back in six months or less.**
  (National Center for Health Statistics)

- **1/3 of adults in this country are constantly dieting and trying to find ways to lose up to five or ten pounds of weight.**
  (International Food Information Council)

- **Many people aged 40 to 80 years old can experience a decreased resting metabolic rate of 25-30%, resulting in automatic weight gain.**
  (Miriam Nelson, Ph.D., Director of the Physical Center for Activity and Nutrition)

- **The craving for high-calorie comfort foods can be caused by lack of sleep.**
  (WebMD)

- **Americans spend $60 billion or more each year in an attempt to lose weight.**
  (US News and World Report)

Natural Weight Loss: The Details

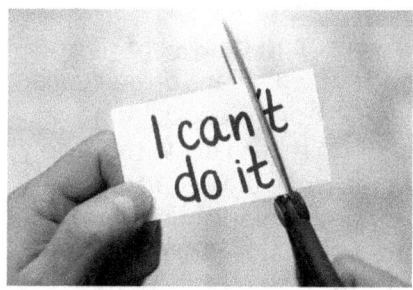

Most weight loss "secrets" are common sense, though there are a few counter-intuitive ideas that can make a BIG difference. Read on so you can get on the road to healthy permanent weight loss.

Uncommon Tip #1: Lose Weight While Watching TV

It's true, you can lose weight watching TV. Just get up off that couch and run in place during the commercials. For a two-hour watching period you can burn off 270 calories. That can be 28 pounds a year. At work you can at least stand instead of sit which research shows for an eight-hour day can help you use up 163 more calories.
(Prevention Magazine)

Uncommon Tip #2: Stress Less, Lose More

Cortisol is a hormone that is produced by stress and anxiety. It also signals the body to store fat, usually as belly fat. If you can reduce your stress with methods such as yoga or walking or meditation, you may find your belly fat will melt away.

Uncommon Tip #3: Chew More, Eat Less

Chewing triggers peptide hormones in the intestines that suppress appetite. One study showed participants chewing a bite of food forty times ate around 12% less than those chewing only fifteen times.
(Joslin Diabetes Center and Harvard Medical School)

Uncommon Tip #4: Eat by Your Body's Clock

According to research by Dr. Norman Cousins, cells are busy with building and repairing, as well as assimilating nutrients from 8 pm in the evening until noon the next day. Between noon and 8 pm, the body is geared toward digestion and metabolism. To get the most from your food and burn as many calories as possible, eat your biggest meals from noon to 8 pm. From noon until 8 in the evening, your cells are ready to digest, which implies that your body will store less fat and digest more fuel.

Uncommon Tip #5: The Power of Castor Oil Packs

One way to lose weight around your waist and belly is to get rid of the "muffin top" or "beer belly," both of which are often caused by undigested food in your intestines. Castor oil packs, done on a regular basis, help your body get rid of all that toxic waste. Apply a castor oil pack to your abdominal area once a week for a month. This is an Edgar Cayce remedy and it works wonders. You'll be surprised at what comes out your back end, so to speak. You can buy complete castor oil pack kits at most health food stores or at the Heritage store online. Instructions can be found in the *Resources* section of this book.

Uncommon Tip #6: Eat Chocolate

According to Dr. Craig A. Maxwell, one delicious way to lose weight is to eat chocolate, specifically dark chocolate, preferably organic with 65% cacao or more... in moderation, of course! This type of chocolate has a type of antioxidant called catechins, which is one type of flavonoid. This type of antioxidant can help increase metabolism, provide extra energy, and reduce cortisol. Cortisol is a stress hormone that, among other things, leads to belly fat. Dark chocolate also has PEA (short for phenylethylamine), which is a naturally occurring substance in the human body that is linked to energy, mood, and attention. It is a vital part of your brain function and is responsible for feelings of pleasure as well as mental acuity. Feeling good is definitely helpful for weight loss!

Get Your Free Consult on Natural Weight Loss & Learn More about Healthy Lifestyles

Visit gohealth.tips/consult to get your free Natural Weight Loss Consult from Prosperity-Abounds.

Common Sense Weight Loss Tips

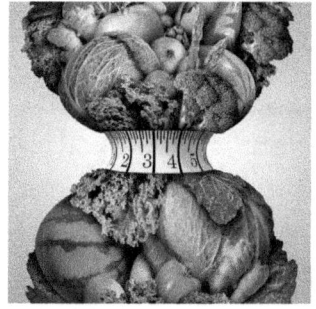

In addition to the previous tips, you can also experience healthy weight loss with the following common-sense tips. These tips can help you lose weight, keep it off, and prevent "yo-yo" weight cycles.

Common Sense Tip #1: Reduce Calories, Increase Exercise

For permanent weight loss, a healthy goal is to lose around one to two pounds a week. Katherine Tallmadge, R.D., weight loss counselor, says eating a healthy diet and getting lots of exercise can help you safely lose at least three pounds a week. You can lose one to two pounds a week just by burning off 500 calories more than you ingest each day.

Common Sense Tip #2: Not All Calories are the Same

Avoid sugar and starch from carbohydrates, especially simple carbohydrates, as much as possible, since these carbs are more likely to be stored as fat (as compared to protein). Insulin is the hormone mainly responsible for fat being stored in the body and sugary and starchy foods cause insulin secretion. When insulin levels are lower it is easier for the body to burn fats and shed pounds.

Common Sense Tip #3: Eat and Drink Before Your Meal

Drink a glass of water (up to 16 ounces) plus a few fiber pills before you begin eating. This will help you feel fuller before eating your meal, allowing you to feel fuller sooner and eat less. Drinking water throughout the day helps you feel fuller which keeps you from eating between meals. Drinking before you exercise releases hormones that help in muscle building (which helps you get the most out of your exercise regimen). Adding probiotics and enzymes will also help increase the efficiency of your digestion (check out gohealth.tips/digestion).

Common Sense Tip #4: Use Nutrition to Boost Weight Loss

Scientists have discovered that taking high-quality whole food supplements can help the body lose weight more easily. For instance, taking AFA bluegreen algae supplements can give the body the important vitamins, minerals, and other micronutrients it needs without adding extra calories (see gohealth.tips/AFA). AFA has been found to support weight loss since a well-nourished body is less likely to crave unhealthy foods, has extra energy for activity, and tends to promote a positive mood. Since AFA is high in chlorophyll, which works on the intestinal lining to enhance the digestion and assimilation of foods, it also helps provide nourishment on a cellular level. Add in high quality probiotic and enzyme supplements (check out "daily packs" that have it all at gohealth.tips/daily) and your digestive system will help your body absorb maximum nutrients.

> ### All-Natural Supplements for Weight Loss Support
>
> **www.Prosperity-Abounds.com**
> **1-866-384-4461 (toll free)**
>
> **Enzymes** (improves digestion, helps reduce weight from undigested food)
> **Probiotics** (acidophilus, bifidus, and full-spectrum varieties to increase digestive effectiveness, reduce cravings)
>
> **Get Enzymes and Probiotics at** gohealth.tips/digestion
>
> **Healthy Snack Bars** (nutrient-rich snack bars that fuel the body during weight loss)
>
> **Get Healthy Snack Bars at** gohealth.tips/bars

Common Sense Tip #5: Get a Diet Plan and a Buddy

Having a reasonable diet plan that improves your eating habits in baby steps has proven more efficient for many people. One study (*Prevention*) reported twice as much weight loss for those keeping a food journal versus those that didn't. After you have taken a little time to study what, how, and when you currently eat, start your plan by making goals that are easy to achieve. In other words, have a long-term goal but break it down into baby steps. Research reported in the Annals of Behavioral Medicine found that making one small permanent change in diet or exercise resulted in losing two times as much belly fat, experiencing a two-and-a-half-inch difference from the waistline, and having quadruple the weight loss over four months. Also consider getting a weight loss buddy or group to help you stay motivated. A study in *Obesity* reports that joining a weight loss group can help participants lose as much as 20% more weight than just dieting alone.

Bonus Tips for Natural Weight Loss

Too Busy? Try This:

If you are a busy person, chances are that you often skip meals or eat on the run. No worries... you can still lose weight with these tips:

- **Snack Healthy**: Try a healthy snack bar instead of a candy bar. Most health bars have pectin and other nutrients that provide soluble fiber, which helps keep blood sugar levels stable and prevents fat from being stored in the body (check out gohealth.tips/bars).
- **Try the Blue Plate Special**: Studies have shown that eating food on a plate that is a different color than your food reduces intake. Ask for a smaller plate to reduce the chances of overeating.
- **Maximize Veggies and Lean Protein:** Even if you have to eat on the run, most fast food joints now offer healthy wraps and salads with calorie counts. Pick the healthiest choice with the least calories.

Prevent the Yo-Yo Diet Effect

Research reports that 95% of dieters gain back the weight they had lost. Use these tips to avoid that.

- **Eat Fat**: Johns Hopkins University reported that people consuming a diet with lots of monounsaturated fats lost small amounts of weight and took fewer days to lose weight than those on diets with lots of carbohydrates. Good sources of these fats are avocados, nuts, olives and oils, such as olive, sunflower, and grapeseed.
- **Eat Enough**: Eating too little can actually slow the metabolism. If you are over age 40, and have trouble losing weight, eat meals of about 400 calories and eat to until full (Dan Benardot, Ph.D., R.D.). Eat no less than 1,200

calories per day or your body will go into starvation mode, and store even more fat (Michael Dansinger, M.D.).

- **Change Your Thinking:** People who lose weight and keep it off don't do crash diets. They tend to be controlled, methodical, and disciplined. They also add one or more new practices, such as yoga or meditation, or even walking to change habits (Inga Treitler, Ph.D.).

Natural Weight Loss at Work

"For years I have been fighting the extra 5 to 10 pounds that I gained after age 40. No matter what I did I could not seem to get rid of those pesky pounds. Using some unusual strategies (eating by the clock and using castor oil packs), and taking some nutritional supplements, really helped tipped the scales. I have lost seven pounds and kept it off for a year and a half. I am delighted!"

~ Joy Herman, Beaufort, SC

Natural Weight Loss Success Profile

Profile: Jackson Lee, age 47

Goal: Lose the "middle age" 20-pound weight gain, especially the beer belly

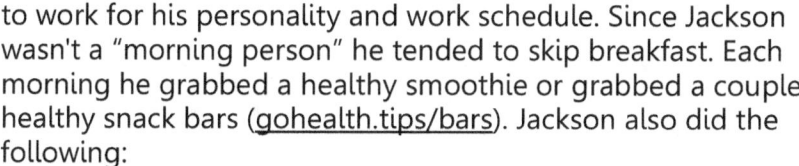

Strategy for Success: Jackson created a weight loss plan most likely to work for his personality and work schedule. Since Jackson wasn't a "morning person" he tended to skip breakfast. Each morning he grabbed a healthy smoothie or grabbed a couple healthy snack bars (gohealth.tips/bars). Jackson also did the following:

- **Yoga**: He started doing a 10-minute yoga workout every day to calm his body and mind, especially when he craved comfort food.
- **Eat the Best of Bad Food**: He researched menus of fast food restaurants where he often ate, and started ordering the healthiest low-calorie options.
- **Shop Smart**: Jackson shopped at the grocery store for lean protein, foods with monounsaturated fats, and some dark chocolate to satisfy "cravings."
- **Simple Exercise:** He took a brisk walk for 15 minutes a day whenever possible. In bad weather, Jackson walked in shopping malls.
- **Nutritional Supplements**: Since he often ate at fast food restaurants, he wanted to be sure his body was getting enough whole food vitamins, minerals, and trace minerals. He took a daily "full spectrum" nutritional packet that contained probiotic and enzymes plus AFA algae, all of which provided a nutritional foundation and improved his digestion (see gohealth.tips/daily).

Results: Over an 18-month period, Jackson succeeded in losing the extra 20 pounds. He did experience some yo-yo weight issues a few times during stressful periods. However, with persistence and patience, Jackson even lost his "beer belly"!

Frequently Asked Questions About Natural Weight Loss

What is a healthy weight for me?
Body Mass Index (BMI) is a good way to determine a healthy weight range for your height (for adults 20 years of age and older). For children, BMI is determined according not just by height and weight, but also by age and sex. You can find many BMI calculators online. Most medical professionals follow these guidelines about BMI:

- Underweight = <18.5
- Normal weight = 18.5–24.9
- Overweight = 25–29.9
- Obesity = BMI of 30 or greater

Using such a calculator, you might determine, for instance, that a healthy weight for a 5' 3" person ranges from 107 to 145 pounds (National Institutes of Health).

How much water should I drink for weight loss?
Did you know that most people are dehydrated, and that drinking even 1% more water can increase your weight loss? Water increases your metabolism, can help you eat less (drink a glass of water before each meal), and can help your body get rid of waste. According to Trent Nessler, P.T., D.P.T., M.P.T., managing director of Baptist Sports Medicine in Nashville, "In general, you should try to drink between half an ounce and an ounce of water for each pound you weigh, every day." So a 170 pound person would need to drink between 65 and 170 ounces of water daily. Drink more if you exercise heavily.

What is your simplest weight loss plan for 20 to 40 pounds of weight loss?
Follow a few simple tips to help you lose weight at a healthy rate:

- Create a weight loss strategy that includes your plans for exercise, types of food you will eat, whether you will stay motivated with a buddy or a structured program, etc.
- Drink enough water, as detailed previously.
- Add one way to increase your weekly exercise (even if it means jogging in place during commercial breaks in a two-hour TV segment) or a 15-minute brisk walk at lunch.
- Choose two to three foods to drop from your diet.
- Write down everything related your strategy: what you eat, how much exercise you do, how much water you drink, and anything else in your weight loss plan.
- Don't deprive yourself. Try something like carb-cycling or eating dark chocolate to keep cravings in check.

What should I do if I wreck my diet?
Don't punish yourself if you give into your cravings. Just note it in your journal, and note any "triggers" that may have caused you to fall off your weight loss plan. Focus on avoiding those triggers in the future. Also, allow yourself a "cheater" day every 10 to 14 days so you avoid sabotaging your plan. Staying hopeful and determined is much more useful than criticizing yourself for having a bad day.

Once I reach my ideal weight, how do I maintain it? Will I have to diet forever?
One of the biggest reason people fail to lose weight is because they "go on a diet" instead of moving into a healthier lifestyle. Once you reach your ideal weight, try some of these additional tips to stay at that weight:
- Sip water throughout the day, stay hydrated, and drink a glass of water before each meal.
- Keep healthy snacks handy, and eat smaller healthy meals frequently rather than eating three large meals. Eat your biggest meal between noon and eight pm.
- Stay faithful to your exercise program. You might even set a goal, such as completing a 5K fun walk/run to stay motivated.

Resources: Castor Oil Packs for Natural Weight Loss

Castor Oil Packs come from intuitive healer Edgar Cayce. These packs are useful for weight loss because they clean the organs of assimilation and elimination. This also clears out the undigested food in the gut, which contributes to the "beer belly" or "muffin top."

1. You will need a wool pack, a quart jar, castor oil, baking soda, an oven-safe dish, a heating pad, a trash bag, two towels, and two washcloths. All can be ordered online or found in health food stores.

2. Fold the pack so it will fit in the bottom of your baking dish. Saturate the pack with castor oil and then warm in oven or toaster oven (no microwave – ever!) Do not wash the wool pack despite the directions that may come with the wool pack.

3. Remove the cloth cover from heating pad, plug in the pad, and turn it on high.

4. Put down a plastic sheet or large trash bag where pack is to be done to protect sofa or bed, positioning the bag so that castor oil will not leak onto the back and flat surface of the sofa or bed.

5. Fold an old towel lengthwise and put on top of plastic so sitting on the plastic bag is more comfortable.

6. Sit comfortably on the towel on the bed or sofa. Place the warmed pack on your abdomen, and put the heating pad over the wool pack. Use another towel to wrap around the heating pad and wool pad, tucking the ends behind you. Optionally wrap a belt around your abdomen to keep the pack in close contact with your abdomen.

7. Leave pack on for 1.5 hours. While pack is on, listen to soft, harmonious music, or read (or be read to) spiritual or

uplifting material. Avoid chaos or negative energy, which could lessen the positive results.

8. After 1.5 hours, remove the pack and store it in the oven-proof dish in a cool dark place.

9. Mix the baking soda with warm water in the quart jar to create a slurry.

10. Wet one of the washcloths and dip it into the baking soda mix. Use the washcloth to scrub the entire area with baking soda. This removes any remaining oil and, more importantly, neutralizes the acids that are pulled out by the pack, transforming them into harmless salts to be flushed out by the lymphatic system.

11. Use another washcloth to clean the baking soda off your abdomen.

12. Other notes: The pack is best done in the evening, prior to bedtime, since this is a very relaxing time. The wool pack is generally folded in half when applied to the body. It is not necessary to wash the pack. Do not share the pack with anyone else.

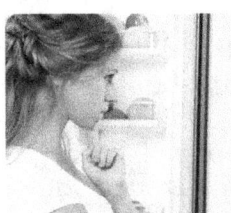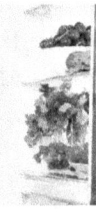

Weight Loss Hacks from Real People

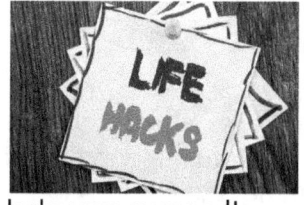

Nothing leads to success like success. In the following section you will find weight loss hacks that helped people just like you succeed in natural weight loss. Look through these tips and tricks, and see if any of them might fit your lifestyle and help you succeed!

Eat a bigger lunch and don't eat dinner

"I used to eat the way most working people do. I would skip breakfast, eat junk food on the run for lunch, and then binge on a huge meal at dinner. As a result, I didn't have enough energy in the morning, had an afternoon "slump" from the junk food lunch, and then gained weight because I ate so much at dinner. I gave my body the most calories when I was least active—when I was sleeping! To lose weight, I decided to change the size of each meal. Instead of just drinking coffee for breakfast, I ate a bagel or yogurt or boiled eggs. I made sure to take time to treat myself to a healthy lunch (healthy sandwich or getting takeout from a salad bar) that was big enough to "stick to my ribs" for the rest of the day. I made sure my lunch had plenty of protein, complex carbs, and some fats. Then I quit eating dinner twice a week. After a few weeks I started skipping dinner three or four days a week. When I reached my desired weight, I skipped dinner just once or twice a week. Now, if my weight increases, I just skip one or two more dinners per week. I am amazed at how this simple strategy helped me lose 48 pounds in 18 months!"
~ Ross K., Garland, TX

Exercise before and after meals

"My doctor told me that if I exercised lightly before and after my biggest meal, I would lose weight faster. Apparently doing even a short 10-minute cardio kick-boxing before a meal activates my body to burn more fat during the workout and throughout the

day. My doctor explained that taking a 15-minute walk after my biggest meal prevented an insulin spike (responsible for fat storage), so I would "work off" the extra calories from meal instead of storing more fat. I tried these short bouts of exercise before and after lunch, and I was so surprised! I lost that stubborn 12 pounds over a four-month period. I love this strategy because it's simple and effective!"
~ Kathryn B., Riverside, CA

Stretch to get the most out of your weight loss plan

"When I started working out at my local gym, I had a few sessions with a personal trainer. In addition to designing a weight loss fitness program for me, she suggested that I attend a yoga class twice a week. Apparently stretching and flexibility maximize the weight loss results from other kinds of exercise. I was willing to try it because my previous fitness strategies did not help me lose as much weight as I wanted. After five months of following my fitness program, I am happy to report that I lost about 15 pounds. Even better, my body feels great and looks great. I move so much better and my workouts are so much easier to power through!"
~ Dennis A., Boise, ID

Pick a Plan... Any Plan!

"Between my full-time job, three kids, aging parents, and busy social schedule, losing weight was impossible! Having failed to shed my extra pounds using every weight loss fad that came around, I was frustrated. Luckily, I met a naturopath who told me that most of her clients failed at weight loss because they did not have a plan that fit their lifestyle. Her clients who were most successful at permanent weight loss followed a plan custom-designed for their schedules and preferences. She offered me three separate weight loss plans. They were simple, designed to fit into my busy life, and required no drastic changes. I chose a plan that focused on short periods of exercise and stretching, small changes to my meals and snacks, and intermittent fasting. I am happy to report that I am now back to my "happy weight," having lost 35 pounds and kept it off for more than a year!"
~ Juliet T., Wilmington, DE

Give in to cravings... just a little

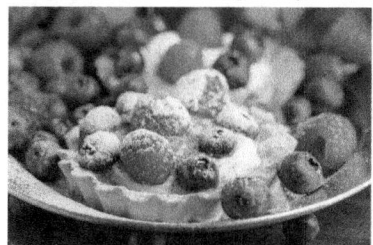

"I am a nutritionist, and one of the ways that I help clients lose weight is to help them with their cravings for sweets. It's natural to crave sweets because sugar causes our bodies to generate 'feel good' neurotransmitters. I give my clients several strategies to use when they have cravings. These strategies help fulfill the craving without wrecking the whole weight loss plan! One, eat a candy bar, just choose the snack size. Two, mix the healthy with the unhealthy, such as eating a handful of nuts with a piece of dark chocolate. Three, go take a walk, which both acts as a distraction and actually reduces hunger. Four, chew some gum or eat some fruit—both of which will satisfy the need for sweets without adding a ton of calories. Five, eat small meals more frequently, especially if you are under stress. This will keep your body from going into what I call the 'stressed starvation mode.' Using all of these strategies has helped many of my clients stick to their weight loss plans and avoid giving into cravings."
~ Joline S., Eastport, MI

Prepare for pitfalls

"I consider myself a 'professional dieter,' and I feel like I have been on some kind of diet since I was a teenager. After years of trying to lose weight and keep it off, I have learned a lot about how to successfully have the body I want. One of the biggest secrets for staying at my desired weight is to prepare for my personal pitfalls... pitfalls are anything that would cause me to make poor choices, and gain weight as a result. I have several major pitfalls, and I prepare for every one of them. For instance, when I'm stressed at work, I tend to crave junk food. I feel like I need to reward and comfort myself with junk food because I am working so hard. I also work long hours, and tend to skip workouts. To prepare for this pitfall, I keep a variety of snacks in the break room—either mini-packs of cookies with less than 100 calories, or healthy food in larger quantities (yogurt, trail mix, fruit and veggies, or sugar free popsicles). My agreement with

myself is that I am allowed to eat one snack when I feel stressed. If I am still not satisfied, I have to 'earn' another snacks by doing a short workout in the company gym (10 to 15 minutes) and drink a bottle of water. I usually find that I don't need a third snack because exercise and water both dampen my appetite. I prepare the same way for every one of my pitfalls. It may sound complex, but it has worked for me for years!"
~ Yolanda R., Santa Fe, NM

Record it or it didn't happen...
"It amazes me how my memory is so bad when it comes to diet and exercise. Every time I have wanted to lose weight, I find that I don't remember everything I have eaten, how much water I have been drinking, and how little exercise I have done. Luckily, I can now use the magic of apps. Using my favorite app, I record everything that goes in my mouth, from a single grape to a full dinner at a popular restaurant. I am always amazed at how fast the calories add up! I set my app to alert me when I have eaten more than half of my allotted calories for the day. My app also reminds me to drink water, counts my steps, and tells me when I still need more exercise. I also connect with other people via the app, and we act as cheerleaders for each other. My success at losing weight and keeping it off is so much better thanks to the wonderful technology of my weight loss app!"
~ Vance W., Austin, NV

Keeping weight off after the diet
"I was one of the 80% of people who failed to keep weight off long term after dieting. After doing the yo-yo diet thing for a while, I decided to learn more about why I could not keep weight off. The most important thing I learned is that for weight loss to be permanent, my plan for losing the weight had to be more about changing my lifestyle habits than about using willpower to resist temptation for a few months. Healthy eating and exercise habits helped me lose weight. Once I got to my ideal weight, I just backed off of my exercise plan some (workouts four days a week instead of five), and allowed myself a few more calories per day (about 200 calories). With this kind of gentle tapering, I have managed to stay at my ideal weight for the last four years!"
~ Samantha H., Riley, KY

Improving digestion for better weight loss

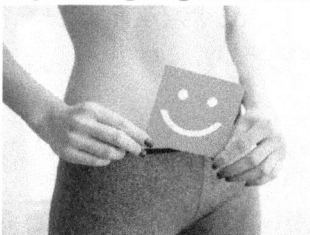

"As a nutritional consultant, when my clients want to lose weight my first questions are about the efficiency of their digestion. The majority of people suffer from poor digestion, which prevents them from absorbing nutrients from food or supplements. Poor digestion also causes a lot of food to get stuck in the digestive tract, and actually ferment. Did you know that a beer belly is really more of a giant chunk of undigested food, which is actually toxic? One of the best weight loss hacks I use is to clean up the digestive system by starting clients on probiotics (acidophilus and bifidus), adding more fiber to their diet, and making sure they are drinking enough water. Clients actually start losing weight with this protocol right away."
~ Renee S., Barnesville, MD

Supplement for all day energy

"When I really got serious about losing some weight and getting fit, I decided to train for a half-marathon. I started eating healthy and exercising hard. A few months into this program, I started feeling really tired all the time. When I asked my personal coach for help, he suggested that I add some wholefood and nutritional supplements that would give me all-day energy, and help my body recover. The major supplements included Coenzyme Q10, bluegreen algae, branch chain amino acids, a mix of proteolytic enzymes, and powdered medicinal mushrooms. With the help of these supplements I started to feel energized rather than drained by my workouts. I also lost more weight than I anticipated, and I got really fit!"
~ Charles B., Bellerose, NY

Decide which part of me is hungry!

"In my quest to lose weight on a permanent basis, one of the most important questions I learned to ask myself is, 'Which part of me is really hungry—my stomach or my tongue?' More times than not, my tongue is the one craving sweets and eats. I have learned to satisfy my tongue with gum, sugar free hard candy, a low-calorie chai latte, or a piece of fruit sweetened with

honey. Once I learned not to give in to my tongue's cravings, I have lost weight (and kept it off) a lot more easily!"
~ Bill K., Virginia Beach, VA

Eat when I am hungry, not tired!
"As weird as this sounds, ever since I was a little kid I could not tell the difference between being hungry and being tired. I have always reached for food whenever I was hungry or tired, so I was chubby when I was younger. As I got older and started working long hours at my job, I ate more and more, and got heavier and heavier. I didn't even realize I ate when I was tired. I really needed sleep more than I needed food. With the help of a support group I was able to analyze my behaviors. Today, I eat when I am hungry, and *only* when I am hungry!"
~ Karen B., Durham, NC

Keep making small tweaks
"When my excess weight became a major health risk, I had to take action. It was all so overwhelming so I decided to take small steps. Every month I would pick one or two tiny aspects of my lifestyle to change... and I do mean tiny! For instance, one month I started eating only one candy bar instead of two every day. I also started drinking a glass of water before each meal. That's it. I didn't start exercising because, quite frankly, I was too heavy to make it possible. But by sticking to every single tweak I made, every month I felt better month by month. That meant each month I could make more significant tweaks with greater impact. By the sixth month, I was able to walk around my office building for 10 minutes during lunch. It may not sound like a lot, but for me it was a miracle. I had not exercised daily for years, so it felt great to walk with ease. I have lost half the weight I want to lose so I have a long way to go, but I keep making those life tweaks that I can handle, and losing weight.
~ Georgeanne B., Riverside, CA

Get Your Free
Weight Loss Consult

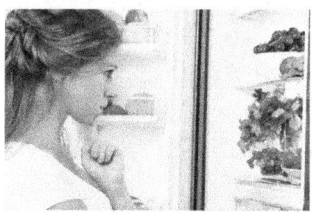

About the Author

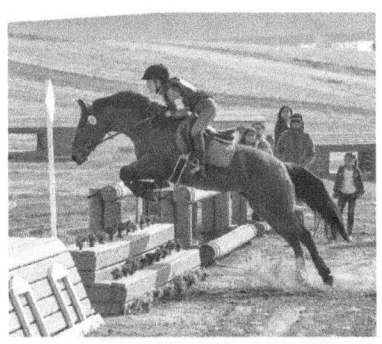

Stephanie Yeh has been researching, learning, and publishing about natural health solutions for over 20 years. Her interests include the use of whole foods, natural supplements, herbs, flower essences, homeopathics, vibrational healing, Edgar Cayce remedies, and bodywork for people and animals.

She has partnered with a wide variety of people to create vibrant natural health for people and their pets.

Stephanie is super passionate about horses and their health, and has enjoyed helping many rescued equines regain health and happiness.

Stephanie enjoys sharing her knowledge of natural healing through a variety of channels, including:

Website: www.Prosperity-Abounds.com

Blog: Prosperity-Abounds.Blogspot.com

Nutritional Consultations: gohealth.tips/consult